PRESCRIPTION FOR HEALTH

HEALTH

from the

TV DOCS

ISBN-13: 978-1514812235
ISBN-10: 1514812231

How to Use This Journal

This journal can be used as a companion while watching your favorite TV Doctor shows. It provides a place for you to keep all of your notes compiled and later use as a reference point about various health topics. The index pages in the back of the book will help you organize all of your notes and information by topic.

Name of TV Show, Episode #, Date of Airing

Show:_____ Episode #:_____ Date:_____

Uses for Apple Cider Vinegar
  Detox Bath - 1c. ACV, 2c. Epsom Salts, lavendar oil
  Clear Stuffy Nose - 1 tea. ACV in glass of water
  Soothe sunburned skin
  Use to clean fresh fruits & veggies

Build A Better Salad
  Vegetarian Protein - Beans
  Omega 3s - Nuts
  MUFAs - Avocado
  Grains - Quinoa

Each page has room for your notes on the various topics covered during each episode.

For more information, visit www.variouswebsite.net

My Rx – Write down something you learned that you can begin to take action on today.

My Rx lose weight to reduce my risk for breast cancer.

This Journal Belongs to:

_____

Shows: _____

Dates: _____

If misplaced, please contact:

Email: _____

Phone: _____

My

R̥

Show:_____ Episode #:_____ Date:_____

My
Rx

My
R℞

My
℞

Show:_____ Episode #:_____ Date:_____

My Rx

Show:_____ Episode #:_____ Date:_____

Show:_____ Episode #:_____ Date:_____

My
Rx

My
Rx

My
R℞

My
Rx

My
Rx

My
Rx

My
R

My
R x

My
R

My

R

Show:_____ Episode #:_____ Date:_____

My
℞

My
R

My
Rx

Show:_____ Episode #:_____ Date:_____

My
Rx

Show:_____ Episode #:_____ Date:_____

My Rx

Show:_____ Episode #:_____ Date:_____

My
R&

Show:_____ Episode #:_____ Date:_____

My Rx

My
R℞

My
Rx

Show:_____ Episode #:_____ Date:_____

My
R

Show:_____ Episode #:_____ Date:_____

My Rx

Show:_____ Episode #:_____ Date:_____

My Rx

My
Rx

My **R̟** _____

My
Rx

Show:_____ Episode #:_____ Date:_____

My
Rx

My
R
x

My
Rx

My
Rx

My
R𝗑

My
R_x

Show:_____ Episode #:_____ Date:_____

My Rx

My
R℈

My
R

My
Rx

My
R

My
R

My
Rx

My
Rx

My
Rx

My Rx

My
R

My
Rx

My
R

My
Rx

My
Rx

My
R

My
R

My
Rx

My
Rx

Show:_____ Episode #:_____ Date:_____

My
R⁢x

My
R

My
Rx

My
R̥

Show:_____ Episode #:_____ Date:_____

My Rx

My
Rx

My
R̶x̶

Show:_____ Episode #:_____ Date:_____

My
Rx

Show:_____ Episode #:_____ Date:_____

My
Rx

Show:_____ Episode #:_____ Date:_____

My
Rx

My
℞

Show:_____ Episode #:_____ Date:_____

My
Rx

Show:_____ Episode #:_____ Date:_____

My Rx

My
Rx _____

Show:_____ Episode #:_____ Date:_____

My Rx

My
R℞

My
Rx

My

R_x

My
R₂

My
R
x

My Rx

My
Rx

My
Rx

Show:_____ Episode #:_____ Date:_____

My
Rx

My
R℘

Show:_____ Episode #:_____ Date:_____

My
Rx

My Rx

My Rx

Show:_____ Episode #:_____ Date:_____

My
Rx

Show:_____ Episode #:_____ Date:_____

My **Rx**

My
R℣

My
Rx

My
Rx

Show:_____ Episode #:_____ Date:_____

My Rx _____

Show:_____ Episode #:_____ Date:_____

My
R℞

My R_____

My
R𝓍

My
R̶x̶

INDEX

INDEX

INDEX

Topic   Page

INDEX

Topic	Page

www.ingramcontent.com/pod-product-compliance
Lightning Source LLC
Chambersburg PA
CBHW070749290526
45795CB00002B/536